I0423075

All

My Fitness

Needs

So this book is for everything:

- Weight
- Measurements
- Grocery lists
- New Menu Ideas
- Workout Ideas
- Feelings/Emotions
- Sleep pattern
- Water intake

(All these things count).

Anything you can think of you can write in this book.

Write everything down in this book. Think of this book like a journal, or like a diary but with a Fitness Twist so more like a Fitness Diary.

DO NOT HOLD BACK

Write down your "Cheats" as well. Everything you write down will help you with your journey.

Remember no one is looking at your diary but you, therefore be honest and true to oneself. Let this book/journal/dairy be your best friend and helper to your goals. Fitness is a journey not a destination. Let it become a lifestyle and not a trend.

Now let's get start! Okay First Things First....

This Book/Journal/Diary is for 8 Weeks

Use it as needed. (Use the days as necessary).
Number your days accordingly. We all know life
happens so if it does, guess what... It's okay. Start
your Day 1 whenever you see fit to do so.
Measurements and weight are located in this Diary
on every entry. You have options so why not
exercise those as well.

But we need to plan. We plan so therefore we do not fail.

So Let's talk Food. What you eat is about 80% of the battle. So
what's the plan?

Look into

- Carb Cycling
- Container counting instead of calories counting
- Paleo Diet
- Vegan Diet
- Smoothie Diet
- Atkins Diet
- Weight Watchers
- Vegetarian Diet

This Journal Belongs to:

Grocery List

New Menu/Recipe Ideas

Day   Date

Weight:

Measurements:

Chest:	Neck:
Left arm:	Right Arm:
Left Forearm:	Right Forearm:
Left Wrist:	Right Wrist:
Waist:	Hips:
Left Thigh:	Right Thigh:
Left Calf:	Right Calf:

Body Mass Index:

Breakfast:

Snack #1:

Lunch:

Snack #2:

Pre-Workout/Post-Workout:

Workout/Length of Workout:

Any weights used during workout? If so, list the weight(s) amount.

Weighted vest/Ankle/Wrist weights/ Waist Trainer?

Dinner:

Vitamins/Supplements:

Water Intake:

How did you sleep last night?

How did you feel today?

How was the workout?

How do you feel after the workout?

Sickness/Illness/ Disease?

Cheats?

Goals:

Day   Date

Weight:

Measurements:

Chest: Neck:

Left arm: Right Arm:

Left Forearm: Right Forearm:

Left Wrist: Right Wrist:

Waist: Hips:

Left Thigh: Right Thigh:

Left Calf: Right Calf:

Body Mass Index:

Breakfast:

Snack #1:

Lunch:

Snack #2:

Pre-Workout/Post-Workout:

Workout/Length of Workout:

Any weights used during workout? If so, list the weight(s) amount.

Weighted vest/Ankle/Wrist weights/ Waist Trainer?

Dinner:

Vitamins/Supplements:

Water Intake:

How did you sleep last night?

How did you feel today?

How was the workout?

How do you feel after the workout?

Sickness/Illness/ Disease?

Cheats?

Goals:

Day   Date

Weight:

Measurements:

Chest: Neck:

Left arm: Right Arm:

Left Forearm: Right Forearm:

Left Wrist: Right Wrist:

Waist: Hips:

Left Thigh: Right Thigh:

Left Calf: Right Calf:

Body Mass Index:

Breakfast:

Snack #1:

Lunch:

Snack #2:

Pre-Workout/Post-Workout:

Workout/Length of Workout:

Any weights used during workout? If so, list the weight(s) amount.

Weighted vest/Ankle/Wrist weights/ Waist Trainer?

Dinner:

Vitamins/Supplements:

Water Intake:

How did you sleep last night?

How did you feel today?

How was the workout?

How do you feel after the workout?

Sickness/Illness/ Disease?

Cheats?

Goals:

Day   Date

Weight:

Measurements:

Chest:	Neck:
Left arm:	Right Arm:
Left Forearm:	Right Forearm:
Left Wrist:	Right Wrist:
Waist:	Hips:
Left Thigh:	Right Thigh:
Left Calf:	Right Calf:

Body Mass Index:

Breakfast:

Snack #1:

Lunch:

Snack #2:

Pre-Workout/Post-Workout:

Workout/Length of Workout:

Any weights used during workout? If so, list the weight(s) amount.

Weighted vest/Ankle/Wrist weights/ Waist Trainer?

Dinner:

Vitamins/Supplements:

Water Intake:

How did you sleep last night?

How did you feel today?

How was the workout?

How do you feel after the workout?

Sickness/Illness/ Disease?

Cheats?

Goals:

Day   Date

Weight:

Measurements:

Chest: Neck:

Left arm: Right Arm:

Left Forearm: Right Forearm:

Left Wrist: Right Wrist:

Waist: Hips:

Left Thigh: Right Thigh:

Left Calf: Right Calf:

Body Mass Index:

Breakfast:

Snack #1:

Lunch:

Snack #2:

Pre-Workout/Post-Workout:

Workout/Length of Workout:

Any weights used during workout? If so, list the weight(s) amount.

Weighted vest/Ankle/Wrist weights/ Waist Trainer?

Dinner:

Vitamins/Supplements:

Water Intake:

How did you sleep last night?

How did you feel today?

How was the workout?

How do you feel after the workout?

Sickness/Illness/ Disease?

Cheats?

Goals:

Day   Date

Weight:

Measurements:

Chest: Neck:

Left arm: Right Arm:

Left Forearm: Right Forearm:

Left Wrist: Right Wrist:

Waist: Hips:

Left Thigh: Right Thigh:

Left Calf: Right Calf:

Body Mass Index:

Breakfast:

Snack #1:

Lunch:

Snack #2:

Pre-Workout/Post-Workout:

Workout/Length of Workout:

Any weights used during workout? If so, list the weight(s) amount.

Weighted vest/Ankle/Wrist weights/ Waist Trainer?

Dinner:

Vitamins/Supplements:

Water Intake:

How did you sleep last night?

How did you feel today?

How was the workout?

How do you feel after the workout?

Sickness/Illness/ Disease?

Cheats?

Goals:

Day   Date

Weight:

Measurements:

Chest: Neck:

Left arm: Right Arm:

Left Forearm: Right Forearm:

Left Wrist: Right Wrist:

Waist: Hips:

Left Thigh: Right Thigh:

Left Calf: Right Calf:

Body Mass Index:

Breakfast:

Snack #1:

Lunch:

Snack #2:

Pre-Workout/Post-Workout:

Workout/Length of Workout:

Any weights used during workout? If so, list the weight(s) amount.

Weighted vest/Ankle/Wrist weights/ Waist Trainer?

Dinner:

Vitamins/Supplements:

Water Intake:

How did you sleep last night?

How did you feel today?

How was the workout?

How do you feel after the workout?

Sickness/Illness/ Disease?

Cheats?

Goals:

Grocery List

New Menu/Recipe Ideas

Day   Date

Weight:

Measurements:

Chest: Neck:

Left arm: Right Arm:

Left Forearm: Right Forearm:

Left Wrist: Right Wrist:

Waist: Hips:

Left Thigh: Right Thigh:

Left Calf: Right Calf:

Body Mass Index:

Breakfast:

Snack #1:

Lunch:

Snack #2:

Pre-Workout/Post-Workout:

Workout/Length of Workout:

Any weights used during workout? If so, list the weight(s) amount.

Weighted vest/Ankle/Wrist weights/ Waist Trainer?

Dinner:

Vitamins/Supplements:

Water Intake:

How did you sleep last night?

How did you feel today?

How was the workout?

How do you feel after the workout?

Sickness/Illness/ Disease?

Cheats?

Goals:

Day   Date

Weight:

Measurements:

Chest:	Neck:
Left arm:	Right Arm:
Left Forearm:	Right Forearm:
Left Wrist:	Right Wrist:
Waist:	Hips:
Left Thigh:	Right Thigh:
Left Calf:	Right Calf:

Body Mass Index:

Breakfast:

Snack #1:

Lunch:

Snack #2:

Pre-Workout/Post-Workout:

Workout/Length of Workout:

Any weights used during workout? If so, list the weight(s) amount.

Weighted vest/Ankle/Wrist weights/ Waist Trainer?

Dinner:

Vitamins/Supplements:

Water Intake:

How did you sleep last night?

How did you feel today?

How was the workout?

How do you feel after the workout?

Sickness/Illness/ Disease?

Cheats?

Goals:

Day   Date

Weight:

Measurements:

Chest: Neck:

Left arm: Right Arm:

Left Forearm: Right Forearm:

Left Wrist: Right Wrist:

Waist: Hips:

Left Thigh: Right Thigh:

Left Calf: Right Calf:

Body Mass Index:

Breakfast:

Snack #1:

Lunch:

Snack #2:

Pre-Workout/Post-Workout:

Workout/Length of Workout:

Any weights used during workout? If so, list the weight(s) amount.

Weighted vest/Ankle/Wrist weights/ Waist Trainer?

Dinner:

Vitamins/Supplements:

Water Intake:

How did you sleep last night?

How did you feel today?

How was the workout?

How do you feel after the workout?

Sickness/Illness/ Disease?

Cheats?

Goals:

Day   Date

Weight:

Measurements:

Chest: Neck:

Left arm: Right Arm:

Left Forearm: Right Forearm:

Left Wrist: Right Wrist:

Waist: Hips:

Left Thigh: Right Thigh:

Left Calf: Right Calf:

Body Mass Index:

Breakfast:

Snack #1:

Lunch:

Snack #2:

Pre-Workout/Post-Workout:

Workout/Length of Workout:

Any weights used during workout? If so, list the weight(s) amount.

Weighted vest/Ankle/Wrist weights/ Waist Trainer?

Dinner:

Vitamins/Supplements:

Water Intake:

How did you sleep last night?

How did you feel today?

How was the workout?

How do you feel after the workout?

Sickness/Illness/ Disease?

Cheats?

Goals:

Day   Date

Weight:

Measurements:

Chest: Neck:

Left arm: Right Arm:

Left Forearm: Right Forearm:

Left Wrist: Right Wrist:

Waist: Hips:

Left Thigh: Right Thigh:

Left Calf: Right Calf:

Body Mass Index:

Breakfast:

Snack #1:

Lunch:

Snack #2:

Pre-Workout/Post-Workout:

Workout/Length of Workout:

Any weights used during workout? If so, list the weight(s) amount.

Weighted vest/Ankle/Wrist weights/ Waist Trainer?

Dinner:

Vitamins/Supplements:

Water Intake:

How did you sleep last night?

How did you feel today?

How was the workout?

How do you feel after the workout?

Sickness/Illness/ Disease?

Cheats?

Goals:

Day   Date

Weight:

Measurements:

Chest:	Neck:
Left arm:	Right Arm:
Left Forearm:	Right Forearm:
Left Wrist:	Right Wrist:
Waist:	Hips:
Left Thigh:	Right Thigh:
Left Calf:	Right Calf:

Body Mass Index:

Breakfast:

Snack #1:

Lunch:

Snack #2:

Pre-Workout/Post-Workout:

Workout/Length of Workout:

Any weights used during workout? If so, list the weight(s) amount.

Weighted vest/Ankle/Wrist weights/ Waist Trainer?

Dinner:

Vitamins/Supplements:

Water Intake:

How did you sleep last night?

How did you feel today?

How was the workout?

How do you feel after the workout?

Sickness/Illness/ Disease?

Cheats?

Goals:

Day   Date

Weight:

Measurements:

Chest: Neck:

Left arm: Right Arm:

Left Forearm: Right Forearm:

Left Wrist: Right Wrist:

Waist: Hips:

Left Thigh: Right Thigh:

Left Calf: Right Calf:

Body Mass Index:

Breakfast:

Snack #1:

Lunch:

Snack #2:

Pre-Workout/Post-Workout:

Workout/Length of Workout:

Any weights used during workout? If so, list the weight(s) amount.

Weighted vest/Ankle/Wrist weights/ Waist Trainer?

Dinner:

Vitamins/Supplements:

Water Intake:

How did you sleep last night?

How did you feel today?

How was the workout?

How do you feel after the workout?

Sickness/Illness/ Disease?

Cheats?

Goals:

Grocery List

New Menu/Recipe Ideas

Day   Date

Weight:

Measurements:

Chest: Neck:

Left arm: Right Arm:

Left Forearm: Right Forearm:

Left Wrist: Right Wrist:

Waist: Hips:

Left Thigh: Right Thigh:

Left Calf: Right Calf:

Body Mass Index:

Breakfast:

Snack #1:

Lunch:

Snack #2:

Pre-Workout/Post-Workout:

Workout/Length of Workout:

Any weights used during workout? If so, list the weight(s) amount.

Weighted vest/Ankle/Wrist weights/ Waist Trainer?

Dinner:

Vitamins/Supplements:

Water Intake:

How did you sleep last night?

How did you feel today?

How was the workout?

How do you feel after the workout?

Sickness/Illness/ Disease?

Cheats?

Goals:

Day   Date

Weight:

Measurements:

Chest: Neck:

Left arm: Right Arm:

Left Forearm: Right Forearm:

Left Wrist: Right Wrist:

Waist: Hips:

Left Thigh: Right Thigh:

Left Calf: Right Calf:

Body Mass Index:

Breakfast:

Snack #1:

Lunch:

Snack #2:

Pre-Workout/Post-Workout:

Workout/Length of Workout:

Any weights used during workout? If so, list the weight(s) amount.

Weighted vest/Ankle/Wrist weights/ Waist Trainer?

Dinner:

Vitamins/Supplements:

Water Intake:

How did you sleep last night?

How did you feel today?

How was the workout?

How do you feel after the workout?

Sickness/Illness/ Disease?

Cheats?

Goals:

Day   Date

Weight:

Measurements:

Chest:	Neck:
Left arm:	Right Arm:
Left Forearm:	Right Forearm:
Left Wrist:	Right Wrist:
Waist:	Hips:
Left Thigh:	Right Thigh:
Left Calf:	Right Calf:

Body Mass Index:

Breakfast:

Snack #1:

Lunch:

Snack #2:

Pre-Workout/Post-Workout:

Workout/Length of Workout:

Any weights used during workout? If so, list the weight(s) amount.

Weighted vest/Ankle/Wrist weights/ Waist Trainer?

Dinner:

Vitamins/Supplements:

Water Intake:

How did you sleep last night?

How did you feel today?

How was the workout?

How do you feel after the workout?

Sickness/Illness/ Disease?

Cheats?

Goals:

Day   Date

Weight:

Measurements:

Chest: Neck:

Left arm: Right Arm:

Left Forearm: Right Forearm:

Left Wrist: Right Wrist:

Waist: Hips:

Left Thigh: Right Thigh:

Left Calf: Right Calf:

Body Mass Index:

Breakfast:

Snack #1:

Lunch:

Snack #2:

Pre-Workout/Post-Workout:

Workout/Length of Workout:

Any weights used during workout? If so, list the weight(s) amount.

Weighted vest/Ankle/Wrist weights/ Waist Trainer?

Dinner:

Vitamins/Supplements:

Water Intake:

How did you sleep last night?

How did you feel today?

How was the workout?

How do you feel after the workout?

Sickness/Illness/ Disease?

Cheats?

Goals:

Day   Date

Weight:

Measurements:

Chest:	Neck:
Left arm:	Right Arm:
Left Forearm:	Right Forearm:
Left Wrist:	Right Wrist:
Waist:	Hips:
Left Thigh:	Right Thigh:
Left Calf:	Right Calf:

Body Mass Index:

Breakfast:

Snack #1:

Lunch:

Snack #2:

Pre-Workout/Post-Workout:

Workout/Length of Workout:

Any weights used during workout? If so, list the weight(s) amount.

Weighted vest/Ankle/Wrist weights/ Waist Trainer?

Dinner:

Vitamins/Supplements:

Water Intake:

How did you sleep last night?

How did you feel today?

How was the workout?

How do you feel after the workout?

Sickness/Illness/ Disease?

Cheats?

Goals:

Day   Date

Weight:

Measurements:

Chest: Neck:

Left arm: Right Arm:

Left Forearm: Right Forearm:

Left Wrist: Right Wrist:

Waist: Hips:

Left Thigh: Right Thigh:

Left Calf: Right Calf:

Body Mass Index:

Breakfast:

Snack #1:

Lunch:

Snack #2:

Pre-Workout/Post-Workout:

Workout/Length of Workout:

Any weights used during workout? If so, list the weight(s) amount.

Weighted vest/Ankle/Wrist weights/ Waist Trainer?

Dinner:

Vitamins/Supplements:

Water Intake:

How did you sleep last night?

How did you feel today?

How was the workout?

How do you feel after the workout?

Sickness/Illness/ Disease?

Cheats?

Goals:

Day   Date

Weight:

Measurements:

Chest:	Neck:
Left arm:	Right Arm:
Left Forearm:	Right Forearm:
Left Wrist:	Right Wrist:
Waist:	Hips:
Left Thigh:	Right Thigh:
Left Calf:	Right Calf:

Body Mass Index:

Breakfast:

Snack #1:

Lunch:

Snack #2:

Pre-Workout/Post-Workout:

Workout/Length of Workout:

Any weights used during workout? If so, list the weight(s) amount.

Weighted vest/Ankle/Wrist weights/ Waist Trainer?

Dinner:

Vitamins/Supplements:

Water Intake:

How did you sleep last night?

How did you feel today?

How was the workout?

How do you feel after the workout?

Sickness/Illness/ Disease?

Cheats?

Goals:

Grocery List

New Menu/Recipe Ideas

Day   Date

Weight:

Measurements:

Chest: Neck:

Left arm: Right Arm:

Left Forearm: Right Forearm:

Left Wrist: Right Wrist:

Waist: Hips:

Left Thigh: Right Thigh:

Left Calf: Right Calf:

Body Mass Index:

Breakfast:

Snack #1:

Lunch:

Snack #2:

Pre-Workout/Post-Workout:

Workout/Length of Workout:

Any weights used during workout? If so, list the weight(s) amount.

Weighted vest/Ankle/Wrist weights/ Waist Trainer?

Dinner:

Vitamins/Supplements:

Water Intake:

How did you sleep last night?

How did you feel today?

How was the workout?

How do you feel after the workout?

Sickness/Illness/ Disease?

Cheats?

Goals:

Day   Date

Weight:

Measurements:

Chest: Neck:

Left arm: Right Arm:

Left Forearm: Right Forearm:

Left Wrist: Right Wrist:

Waist: Hips:

Left Thigh: Right Thigh:

Left Calf: Right Calf:

Body Mass Index:

Breakfast:

Snack #1:

Lunch:

Snack #2:

Pre-Workout/Post-Workout:

Workout/Length of Workout:

Any weights used during workout? If so, list the weight(s) amount.

Weighted vest/Ankle/Wrist weights/ Waist Trainer?

Dinner:

Vitamins/Supplements:

Water Intake:

How did you sleep last night?

How did you feel today?

How was the workout?

How do you feel after the workout?

Sickness/Illness/ Disease?

Cheats?

Goals:

Day   Date

Weight:

Measurements:

Chest: Neck:

Left arm: Right Arm:

Left Forearm: Right Forearm:

Left Wrist: Right Wrist:

Waist: Hips:

Left Thigh: Right Thigh:

Left Calf: Right Calf:

Body Mass Index:

Breakfast:

Snack #1:

Lunch:

Snack #2:

Pre-Workout/Post-Workout:

Workout/Length of Workout:

Any weights used during workout? If so, list the weight(s) amount.

Weighted vest/Ankle/Wrist weights/ Waist Trainer?

Dinner:

Vitamins/Supplements:

Water Intake:

How did you sleep last night?

How did you feel today?

How was the workout?

How do you feel after the workout?

Sickness/Illness/ Disease?

Cheats?

Goals:

Day   Date

Weight:

Measurements:

Chest: Neck:

Left arm: Right Arm:

Left Forearm: Right Forearm:

Left Wrist: Right Wrist:

Waist: Hips:

Left Thigh: Right Thigh:

Left Calf: Right Calf:

Body Mass Index:

Breakfast:

Snack #1:

Lunch:

Snack #2:

Pre-Workout/Post-Workout:

Workout/Length of Workout:

Any weights used during workout? If so, list the weight(s) amount.

Weighted vest/Ankle/Wrist weights/ Waist Trainer?

Dinner:

Vitamins/Supplements:

Water Intake:

How did you sleep last night?

How did you feel today?

How was the workout?

How do you feel after the workout?

Sickness/Illness/ Disease?

Cheats?

Goals:

Day   Date

Weight:

Measurements:

Chest: Neck:

Left arm: Right Arm:

Left Forearm: Right Forearm:

Left Wrist: Right Wrist:

Waist: Hips:

Left Thigh: Right Thigh:

Left Calf: Right Calf:

Body Mass Index:

Breakfast:

Snack #1:

Lunch:

Snack #2:

Pre-Workout/Post-Workout:

Workout/Length of Workout:

Any weights used during workout? If so, list the weight(s) amount.

Weighted vest/Ankle/Wrist weights/ Waist Trainer?

Dinner:

Vitamins/Supplements:

Water Intake:

How did you sleep last night?

How did you feel today?

How was the workout?

How do you feel after the workout?

Sickness/Illness/ Disease?

Cheats?

Goals:

Day   Date

Weight:

Measurements:

Chest: Neck:

Left arm: Right Arm:

Left Forearm: Right Forearm:

Left Wrist: Right Wrist:

Waist: Hips:

Left Thigh: Right Thigh:

Left Calf: Right Calf:

Body Mass Index:

Breakfast:

Snack #1:

Lunch:

Snack #2:

Pre-Workout/Post-Workout:

Workout/Length of Workout:

Any weights used during workout? If so, list the weight(s) amount.

Weighted vest/Ankle/Wrist weights/ Waist Trainer?

Dinner:

Vitamins/Supplements:

Water Intake:

How did you sleep last night?

How did you feel today?

How was the workout?

How do you feel after the workout?

Sickness/Illness/ Disease?

Cheats?

Goals:

Day   Date

Weight:

Measurements:

Chest: Neck:

Left arm: Right Arm:

Left Forearm: Right Forearm:

Left Wrist: Right Wrist:

Waist: Hips:

Left Thigh: Right Thigh:

Left Calf: Right Calf:

Body Mass Index:

Breakfast:

Snack #1:

Lunch:

Snack #2:

Pre-Workout/Post-Workout:

Workout/Length of Workout:

Any weights used during workout? If so, list the weight(s) amount.

Weighted vest/Ankle/Wrist weights/ Waist Trainer?

Dinner:

Vitamins/Supplements:

Water Intake:

How did you sleep last night?

How did you feel today?

How was the workout?

How do you feel after the workout?

Sickness/Illness/ Disease?

Cheats?

Goals:

Grocery List

New Menu/Recipe Ideas

Day   Date

Weight:

Measurements:

Chest: Neck:

Left arm: Right Arm:

Left Forearm: Right Forearm:

Left Wrist: Right Wrist:

Waist: Hips:

Left Thigh: Right Thigh:

Left Calf: Right Calf:

Body Mass Index:

Breakfast:

Snack #1:

Lunch:

Snack #2:

Pre-Workout/Post-Workout:

Workout/Length of Workout:

Any weights used during workout? If so, list the weight(s) amount.

Weighted vest/Ankle/Wrist weights/ Waist Trainer?

Dinner:

Vitamins/Supplements:

Water Intake:

How did you sleep last night?

How did you feel today?

How was the workout?

How do you feel after the workout?

Sickness/Illness/ Disease?

Cheats?

Goals:

Day   Date

Weight:

Measurements:

Chest: Neck:

Left arm: Right Arm:

Left Forearm: Right Forearm:

Left Wrist: Right Wrist:

Waist: Hips:

Left Thigh: Right Thigh:

Left Calf: Right Calf:

Body Mass Index:

Breakfast:

Snack #1:

Lunch:

Snack #2:

Pre-Workout/Post-Workout:

Workout/Length of Workout:

Any weights used during workout? If so, list the weight(s) amount.

Weighted vest/Ankle/Wrist weights/ Waist Trainer?

Dinner:

Vitamins/Supplements:

Water Intake:

How did you sleep last night?

How did you feel today?

How was the workout?

How do you feel after the workout?

Sickness/Illness/ Disease?

Cheats?

Goals:

Day   Date

Weight:

Measurements:

Chest: Neck:

Left arm: Right Arm:

Left Forearm: Right Forearm:

Left Wrist: Right Wrist:

Waist: Hips:

Left Thigh: Right Thigh:

Left Calf: Right Calf:

Body Mass Index:

Breakfast:

Snack #1:

Lunch:

Snack #2:

Pre-Workout/Post-Workout:

Workout/Length of Workout:

Any weights used during workout? If so, list the weight(s) amount.

Weighted vest/Ankle/Wrist weights/ Waist Trainer?

Dinner:

Vitamins/Supplements:

Water Intake:

How did you sleep last night?

How did you feel today?

How was the workout?

How do you feel after the workout?

Sickness/Illness/ Disease?

Cheats?

Goals:

Day   Date

Weight:

Measurements:

Chest: Neck:

Left arm: Right Arm:

Left Forearm: Right Forearm:

Left Wrist: Right Wrist:

Waist: Hips:

Left Thigh: Right Thigh:

Left Calf: Right Calf:

Body Mass Index:

Breakfast:

Snack #1:

Lunch:

Snack #2:

Pre-Workout/Post-Workout:

Workout/Length of Workout:

Any weights used during workout? If so, list the weight(s) amount.

Weighted vest/Ankle/Wrist weights/ Waist Trainer?

Dinner:

Vitamins/Supplements:

Water Intake:

How did you sleep last night?

How did you feel today?

How was the workout?

How do you feel after the workout?

Sickness/Illness/ Disease?

Cheats?

Goals:

Day   Date

Weight:

Measurements:

Chest: Neck:

Left arm: Right Arm:

Left Forearm: Right Forearm:

Left Wrist: Right Wrist:

Waist: Hips:

Left Thigh: Right Thigh:

Left Calf: Right Calf:

Body Mass Index:

Breakfast:

Snack #1:

Lunch:

Snack #2:

Pre-Workout/Post-Workout:

Workout/Length of Workout:

Any weights used during workout? If so, list the weight(s) amount.

Weighted vest/Ankle/Wrist weights/ Waist Trainer?

Dinner:

Vitamins/Supplements:

Water Intake:

How did you sleep last night?

How did you feel today?

How was the workout?

How do you feel after the workout?

Sickness/Illness/ Disease?

Cheats?

Goals:

Day   Date

Weight:

Measurements:

Chest:	Neck:
Left arm:	Right Arm:
Left Forearm:	Right Forearm:
Left Wrist:	Right Wrist:
Waist:	Hips:
Left Thigh:	Right Thigh:
Left Calf:	Right Calf:

Body Mass Index:

Breakfast:

Snack #1:

Lunch:

Snack #2:

Pre-Workout/Post-Workout:

Workout/Length of Workout:

Any weights used during workout? If so, list the weight(s) amount.

Weighted vest/Ankle/Wrist weights/ Waist Trainer?

Dinner:

Vitamins/Supplements:

Water Intake:

How did you sleep last night?

How did you feel today?

How was the workout?

How do you feel after the workout?

Sickness/Illness/ Disease?

Cheats?

Goals:

Day   Date

Weight:

Measurements:

Chest: Neck:

Left arm: Right Arm:

Left Forearm: Right Forearm:

Left Wrist: Right Wrist:

Waist: Hips:

Left Thigh: Right Thigh:

Left Calf: Right Calf:

Body Mass Index:

Breakfast:

Snack #1:

Lunch:

Snack #2:

Pre-Workout/Post-Workout:

Workout/Length of Workout:

Any weights used during workout? If so, list the weight(s) amount.

Weighted vest/Ankle/Wrist weights/ Waist Trainer?

Dinner:

Vitamins/Supplements:

Water Intake:

How did you sleep last night?

How did you feel today?

How was the workout?

How do you feel after the workout?

Sickness/Illness/ Disease?

Cheats?

Goals:

Grocery List

New Menu/Recipe Ideas

Day   Date

Weight:

Measurements:

Chest: Neck:

Left arm: Right Arm:

Left Forearm: Right Forearm:

Left Wrist: Right Wrist:

Waist: Hips:

Left Thigh: Right Thigh:

Left Calf: Right Calf:

Body Mass Index:

Breakfast:

Snack #1:

Lunch:

Snack #2:

Pre-Workout/Post-Workout:

Workout/Length of Workout:

Any weights used during workout? If so, list the weight(s) amount.

Weighted vest/Ankle/Wrist weights/ Waist Trainer?

Dinner:

Vitamins/Supplements:

Water Intake:

How did you sleep last night?

How did you feel today?

How was the workout?

How do you feel after the workout?

Sickness/Illness/ Disease?

Cheats?

Goals:

Day   Date

Weight:

Measurements:

Chest: Neck:

Left arm: Right Arm:

Left Forearm: Right Forearm:

Left Wrist: Right Wrist:

Waist: Hips:

Left Thigh: Right Thigh:

Left Calf: Right Calf:

Body Mass Index:

Breakfast:

Snack #1:

Lunch:

Snack #2:

Pre-Workout/Post-Workout:

Workout/Length of Workout:

Any weights used during workout? If so, list the weight(s) amount.

Weighted vest/Ankle/Wrist weights/ Waist Trainer?

Dinner:

Vitamins/Supplements:

Water Intake:

How did you sleep last night?

How did you feel today?

How was the workout?

How do you feel after the workout?

Sickness/Illness/ Disease?

Cheats?

Goals:

Day   Date

Weight:

Measurements:

Chest: Neck:

Left arm: Right Arm:

Left Forearm: Right Forearm:

Left Wrist: Right Wrist:

Waist: Hips:

Left Thigh: Right Thigh:

Left Calf: Right Calf:

Body Mass Index:

Breakfast:

Snack #1:

Lunch:

Snack #2:

Pre-Workout/Post-Workout:

Workout/Length of Workout:

Any weights used during workout? If so, list the weight(s) amount.

Weighted vest/Ankle/Wrist weights/ Waist Trainer?

Dinner:

Vitamins/Supplements:

Water Intake:

How did you sleep last night?

How did you feel today?

How was the workout?

How do you feel after the workout?

Sickness/Illness/ Disease?

Cheats?

Goals:

Day   Date

Weight:

Measurements:

Chest: Neck:

Left arm: Right Arm:

Left Forearm: Right Forearm:

Left Wrist: Right Wrist:

Waist: Hips:

Left Thigh: Right Thigh:

Left Calf: Right Calf:

Body Mass Index:

Breakfast:

Snack #1:

Lunch:

Snack #2:

Pre-Workout/Post-Workout:

Workout/Length of Workout:

Any weights used during workout? If so, list the weight(s) amount.

Weighted vest/Ankle/Wrist weights/ Waist Trainer?

Dinner:

Vitamins/Supplements:

Water Intake:

How did you sleep last night?

How did you feel today?

How was the workout?

How do you feel after the workout?

Sickness/Illness/ Disease?

Cheats?

Goals:

Day   Date

Weight:

Measurements:

Chest: Neck:

Left arm: Right Arm:

Left Forearm: Right Forearm:

Left Wrist: Right Wrist:

Waist: Hips:

Left Thigh: Right Thigh:

Left Calf: Right Calf:

Body Mass Index:

Breakfast:

Snack #1:

Lunch:

Snack #2:

Pre-Workout/Post-Workout:

Workout/Length of Workout:

Any weights used during workout? If so, list the weight(s) amount.

Weighted vest/Ankle/Wrist weights/ Waist Trainer?

Dinner:

Vitamins/Supplements:

Water Intake:

How did you sleep last night?

How did you feel today?

How was the workout?

How do you feel after the workout?

Sickness/Illness/ Disease?

Cheats?

Goals:

Day   Date

Weight:

Measurements:

Chest: Neck:

Left arm: Right Arm:

Left Forearm: Right Forearm:

Left Wrist: Right Wrist:

Waist: Hips:

Left Thigh: Right Thigh:

Left Calf: Right Calf:

Body Mass Index:

Breakfast:

Snack #1:

Lunch:

Snack #2:

Pre-Workout/Post-Workout:

Workout/Length of Workout:

Any weights used during workout? If so, list the weight(s) amount.

Weighted vest/Ankle/Wrist weights/ Waist Trainer?

Dinner:

Vitamins/Supplements:

Water Intake:

How did you sleep last night?

How did you feel today?

How was the workout?

How do you feel after the workout?

Sickness/Illness/ Disease?

Cheats?

Goals:

Day   Date

Weight:

Measurements:

Chest:	Neck:
Left arm:	Right Arm:
Left Forearm:	Right Forearm:
Left Wrist:	Right Wrist:
Waist:	Hips:
Left Thigh:	Right Thigh:
Left Calf:	Right Calf:

Body Mass Index:

Breakfast:

Snack #1:

Lunch:

Snack #2:

Pre-Workout/Post-Workout:

Workout/Length of Workout:

Any weights used during workout? If so, list the weight(s) amount.

Weighted vest/Ankle/Wrist weights/ Waist Trainer?

Dinner:

Vitamins/Supplements:

Water Intake:

How did you sleep last night?

How did you feel today?

How was the workout?

How do you feel after the workout?

Sickness/Illness/ Disease?

Cheats?

Goals:

Grocery List

New Menu/Recipe Ideas

Day   Date

Weight:

Measurements:

Chest: Neck:

Left arm: Right Arm:

Left Forearm: Right Forearm:

Left Wrist: Right Wrist:

Waist: Hips:

Left Thigh: Right Thigh:

Left Calf: Right Calf:

Body Mass Index:

Breakfast:

Snack #1:

Lunch:

Snack #2:

Pre-Workout/Post-Workout:

Workout/Length of Workout:

Any weights used during workout? If so, list the weight(s) amount.

Weighted vest/Ankle/Wrist weights/ Waist Trainer?

Dinner:

Vitamins/Supplements:

Water Intake:

How did you sleep last night?

How did you feel today?

How was the workout?

How do you feel after the workout?

Sickness/Illness/ Disease?

Cheats?

Goals:

Day   Date

Weight:

Measurements:

Chest:	Neck:
Left arm:	Right Arm:
Left Forearm:	Right Forearm:
Left Wrist:	Right Wrist:
Waist:	Hips:
Left Thigh:	Right Thigh:
Left Calf:	Right Calf:

Body Mass Index:

Breakfast:

Snack #1:

Lunch:

Snack #2:

Pre-Workout/Post-Workout:

Workout/Length of Workout:

Any weights used during workout? If so, list the weight(s) amount.

Weighted vest/Ankle/Wrist weights/ Waist Trainer?

Dinner:

Vitamins/Supplements:

Water Intake:

How did you sleep last night?

How did you feel today?

How was the workout?

How do you feel after the workout?

Sickness/Illness/ Disease?

Cheats?

Goals:

Day   Date

Weight:

Measurements:

Chest: Neck:

Left arm: Right Arm:

Left Forearm: Right Forearm:

Left Wrist: Right Wrist:

Waist: Hips:

Left Thigh: Right Thigh:

Left Calf: Right Calf:

Body Mass Index:

Breakfast:

Snack #1:

Lunch:

Snack #2:

Pre-Workout/Post-Workout:

Workout/Length of Workout:

Any weights used during workout? If so, list the weight(s) amount.

Weighted vest/Ankle/Wrist weights/ Waist Trainer?

Dinner:

Vitamins/Supplements:

Water Intake:

How did you sleep last night?

How did you feel today?

How was the workout?

How do you feel after the workout?

Sickness/Illness/ Disease?

Cheats?

Goals:

Day   Date

Weight:

Measurements:

Chest: Neck:

Left arm: Right Arm:

Left Forearm: Right Forearm:

Left Wrist: Right Wrist:

Waist: Hips:

Left Thigh: Right Thigh:

Left Calf: Right Calf:

Body Mass Index:

Breakfast:

Snack #1:

Lunch:

Snack #2:

Pre-Workout/Post-Workout:

Workout/Length of Workout:

Any weights used during workout? If so, list the weight(s) amount.

Weighted vest/Ankle/Wrist weights/ Waist Trainer?

Dinner:

Vitamins/Supplements:

Water Intake:

How did you sleep last night?

How did you feel today?

How was the workout?

How do you feel after the workout?

Sickness/Illness/ Disease?

Cheats?

Goals:

Day   Date

Weight:

Measurements:

Chest: Neck:

Left arm: Right Arm:

Left Forearm: Right Forearm:

Left Wrist: Right Wrist:

Waist: Hips:

Left Thigh: Right Thigh:

Left Calf: Right Calf:

Body Mass Index:

Breakfast:

Snack #1:

Lunch:

Snack #2:

Pre-Workout/Post-Workout:

Workout/Length of Workout:

Any weights used during workout? If so, list the weight(s) amount.

Weighted vest/Ankle/Wrist weights/ Waist Trainer?

Dinner:

Vitamins/Supplements:

Water Intake:

How did you sleep last night?

How did you feel today?

How was the workout?

How do you feel after the workout?

Sickness/Illness/ Disease?

Cheats?

Goals:

Day   Date

Weight:

Measurements:

Chest: Neck:

Left arm: Right Arm:

Left Forearm: Right Forearm:

Left Wrist: Right Wrist:

Waist: Hips:

Left Thigh: Right Thigh:

Left Calf: Right Calf:

Body Mass Index:

Breakfast:

Snack #1:

Lunch:

Snack #2:

Pre-Workout/Post-Workout:

Workout/Length of Workout:

Any weights used during workout? If so, list the weight(s) amount.

Weighted vest/Ankle/Wrist weights/ Waist Trainer?

Dinner:

Vitamins/Supplements:

Water Intake:

How did you sleep last night?

How did you feel today?

How was the workout?

How do you feel after the workout?

Sickness/Illness/ Disease?

Cheats?

Goals:

Day   Date

Weight:

Measurements:

Chest: Neck:

Left arm: Right Arm:

Left Forearm: Right Forearm:

Left Wrist: Right Wrist:

Waist: Hips:

Left Thigh: Right Thigh:

Left Calf: Right Calf:

Body Mass Index:

Breakfast:

Snack #1:

Lunch:

Snack #2:

Pre-Workout/Post-Workout:

Workout/Length of Workout:

Any weights used during workout? If so, list the weight(s) amount.

Weighted vest/Ankle/Wrist weights/ Waist Trainer?

Dinner:

Vitamins/Supplements:

Water Intake:

How did you sleep last night?

How did you feel today?

How was the workout?

How do you feel after the workout?

Sickness/Illness/ Disease?

Cheats?

Goals:

Grocery List

New Menu/Recipe Ideas

Day   Date

Weight:

Measurements:

Chest: Neck:

Left arm: Right Arm:

Left Forearm: Right Forearm:

Left Wrist: Right Wrist:

Waist: Hips:

Left Thigh: Right Thigh:

Left Calf: Right Calf:

Body Mass Index:

Breakfast:

Snack #1:

Lunch:

Snack #2:

Pre-Workout/Post-Workout:

Workout/Length of Workout:

Any weights used during workout? If so, list the weight(s) amount.

Weighted vest/Ankle/Wrist weights/ Waist Trainer?

Dinner:

Vitamins/Supplements:

Water Intake:

How did you sleep last night?

How did you feel today?

How was the workout?

How do you feel after the workout?

Sickness/Illness/ Disease?

Cheats?

Goals:

Day   Date

Weight:

Measurements:

Chest:	Neck:
Left arm:	Right Arm:
Left Forearm:	Right Forearm:
Left Wrist:	Right Wrist:
Waist:	Hips:
Left Thigh:	Right Thigh:
Left Calf:	Right Calf:

Body Mass Index:

Breakfast:

Snack #1:

Lunch:

Snack #2:

Pre-Workout/Post-Workout:

Workout/Length of Workout:

Any weights used during workout? If so, list the weight(s) amount.

Weighted vest/Ankle/Wrist weights/ Waist Trainer?

Dinner:

Vitamins/Supplements:

Water Intake:

How did you sleep last night?

How did you feel today?

How was the workout?

How do you feel after the workout?

Sickness/Illness/ Disease?

Cheats?

Goals:

Day   Date

Weight:

Measurements:

Chest:	Neck:
Left arm:	Right Arm:
Left Forearm:	Right Forearm:
Left Wrist:	Right Wrist:
Waist:	Hips:
Left Thigh:	Right Thigh:
Left Calf:	Right Calf:

Body Mass Index:

Breakfast:

Snack #1:

Lunch:

Snack #2:

Pre-Workout/Post-Workout:

Workout/Length of Workout:

Any weights used during workout? If so, list the weight(s) amount.

Weighted vest/Ankle/Wrist weights/ Waist Trainer?

Dinner:

Vitamins/Supplements:

Water Intake:

How did you sleep last night?

How did you feel today?

How was the workout?

How do you feel after the workout?

Sickness/Illness/ Disease?

Cheats?

Goals:

Day

Date

Weight:

Measurements:

Chest:	Neck:
Left arm:	Right Arm:
Left Forearm:	Right Forearm:
Left Wrist:	Right Wrist:
Waist:	Hips:
Left Thigh:	Right Thigh:
Left Calf:	Right Calf:

Body Mass Index:

Breakfast:

Snack #1:

Lunch:

Snack #2:

Pre-Workout/Post-Workout:

Workout/Length of Workout:

Any weights used during workout? If so, list the weight(s) amount.

Weighted vest/Ankle/Wrist weights/ Waist Trainer?

Dinner:

Vitamins/Supplements:

Water Intake:

How did you sleep last night?

How did you feel today?

How was the workout?

How do you feel after the workout?

Sickness/Illness/ Disease?

Cheats?

Goals:

Day   Date

Weight:

Measurements:

Chest: Neck:

Left arm: Right Arm:

Left Forearm: Right Forearm:

Left Wrist: Right Wrist:

Waist: Hips:

Left Thigh: Right Thigh:

Left Calf: Right Calf:

Body Mass Index:

Breakfast:

Snack #1:

Lunch:

Snack #2:

Pre-Workout/Post-Workout:

Workout/Length of Workout:

Any weights used during workout? If so, list the weight(s) amount.

Weighted vest/Ankle/Wrist weights/ Waist Trainer?

Dinner:

Vitamins/Supplements:

Water Intake:

How did you sleep last night?

How did you feel today?

How was the workout?

How do you feel after the workout?

Sickness/Illness/ Disease?

Cheats?

Goals:

Day   Date

Weight:

Measurements:

Chest:	Neck:
Left arm:	Right Arm:
Left Forearm:	Right Forearm:
Left Wrist:	Right Wrist:
Waist:	Hips:
Left Thigh:	Right Thigh:
Left Calf:	Right Calf:

Body Mass Index:

Breakfast:

Snack #1:

Lunch:

Snack #2:

Pre-Workout/Post-Workout:

Workout/Length of Workout:

Any weights used during workout? If so, list the weight(s) amount.

Weighted vest/Ankle/Wrist weights/ Waist Trainer?

Dinner:

Vitamins/Supplements:

Water Intake:

How did you sleep last night?

How did you feel today?

How was the workout?

How do you feel after the workout?

Sickness/Illness/ Disease?

Cheats?

Goals:

Day   Date

Weight:

Measurements:

Chest: Neck:

Left arm: Right Arm:

Left Forearm: Right Forearm:

Left Wrist: Right Wrist:

Waist: Hips:

Left Thigh: Right Thigh:

Left Calf: Right Calf:

Body Mass Index:

Breakfast:

Snack #1:

Lunch:

Snack #2:

Pre-Workout/Post-Workout:

Workout/Length of Workout:

Any weights used during workout? If so, list the weight(s) amount.

Weighted vest/Ankle/Wrist weights/ Waist Trainer?

Dinner:

Vitamins/Supplements:

Water Intake:

How did you sleep last night?

How did you feel today?

How was the workout?

How do you feel after the workout?

Sickness/Illness/ Disease?

Cheats?

Goals:

And You're Finish!

You have completed 8 Weeks of your fitness Journey!

There is nothing more refreshing than accomplishing and achieving goals!

Pat yourself on the back….

Keep Going

One more day on me …

Day   Date

Weight:

Measurements:

Chest: Neck:

Left arm: Right Arm:

Left Forearm: Right Forearm:

Left Wrist: Right Wrist:

Waist: Hips:

Left Thigh: Right Thigh:

Left Calf: Right Calf:

Body Mass Index:

Breakfast:

Snack #1:

Lunch:

Snack #2:

Pre-Workout/Post-Workout:

Workout/Length of Workout:

Any weights used during workout? If so, list the amount of weights.

Weighted vest/Ankle/Wrist weights/ Waist Trainer?

Dinner:

Vitamins/Supplements:

Water Intake:

How did you sleep last night?

How did you feel today?

How was the workout?

How do you feel after the workout?

Sickness/Illness/ Disease?

Cheats?

Goals:

Time For

A

New

Diary!

www.ingramcontent.com/pod-product-compliance
Lightning Source LLC
Chambersburg PA
CBHW070110290526
45789CB00005B/1991